# Parenting Daughters in a Perverse World

## *"How to Raise a Successful Woman out of Your Girl Child"*

BY MORGEN ERIC MHLANGA

# Contents

# Introduction

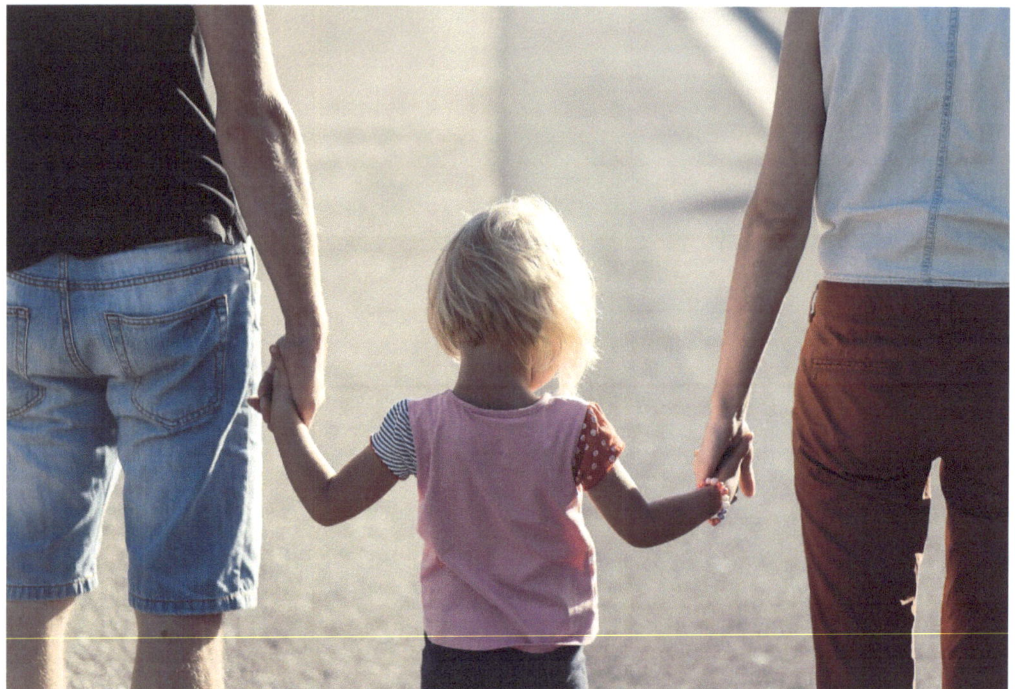



The relationship between parents and daughters is often considered to be one of the most complex and nuanced bonds in the world. From the moment a daughter is born, parents are faced with the unique challenge of guiding their daughters through life while also trying to maintain a close and loving relationship. Throughout the years, parents and daughters will go through a range of emotions, including happiness, frustration, and even anger. But despite all of the ups and downs, there is often a deep and lasting connection between parents and daughters. This connection is often rooted in shared experiences, such as the bond of pregnancy and childbirth, and shared values, such as the importance of family and tradition. Throughout the different stages of a daughter's life, the parent-daughter relationship will change and evolve. But no matter what, parents and daughters often share a deep and unbreakable connection that is unlike any other.

This book will take you through several important subjects such as helping your daughter find her path in life; how to navigate your daughter's teen years; talking to her about sex and relationships; how to encourage a positive self-image and body image; as well as managing disagreements and conflict amongst other subjects.

For example; parenting a teenager can be one of the most challenging and rewarding experiences of a parent's life. Teenagers are in a time of their lives when they are undergoing major physical, emotional, and social changes. They are often trying to find their own identity and place in the world, which can lead to conflict with their parents. During the teenage years, parents may find themselves walking a fine line between giving their daughters the space they need to grow and make their own choices, and providing the guidance and support they need to stay on the right path. It is a time when parents must strike a delicate balance between being a friend and being a parent. It is also a time when parents must learn to accept that their daughters are becoming young women and that they will need to start making their own decisions about their future.

For many parents, one of the most difficult parts of parenting a daughter is letting her find her path in life. It can be hard to watch your daughter make mistakes or take a different path than you envisioned for her. But it is important to remember that your daughter is her own person, with her unique strengths and interests. The best thing you can do is to support her in whatever path she chooses, even if it is not the one you would have chosen for her. You can do this by being an active listener, being available to talk, and not being judgmental. You should also encourage her to pursue her interests and passions and provide her with the resources she needs to succeed. Remember that your daughter's journey is her own, and it is not your job to control it. Instead, your job is to be there for her as she finds her way in the world.

Throughout the stages of your daughter's growth, always maintain an open communication channel. As a parent, you should avoid using accusatory language, and instead try to use "I" statements and active listening. You should also be sure to set a good example by being open and honest with your daughter. If you can keep the lines of communication open you will be able to maintain a close and supportive relationship with your daughter, even as they navigate the challenging years.

Another important aspect of parenting a daughter is establishing healthy boundaries. This means setting clear rules and limits, while still giving your daughter the freedom to make her own choices. For example, you may want to establish rules around curfew or social media use, but you should also give your daughter some flexibility to make her own decisions within those boundaries. It is also important to respect your daughter's privacy, and not to overstep her boundaries by snooping through her things or reading her texts. By establishing healthy boundaries, parents can help their daughters develop a sense of responsibility and independence, while still providing them with the support and guidance they need. It is a delicate balance, but one that is essential for maintaining a healthy and positive relationship.

Conflict and disagreements are a normal and healthy part of any relationship, including the relationship between a parent and a daughter. During the teenage years, these conflicts may be especially pronounced, as daughters often begin to assert their independence and test boundaries. Parents need to approach these conflicts calmly and respectfully and try to see things from their daughter's perspective instead of immediately jumping to conclusions or getting angry. It is also important to remember that sometimes it is okay to just agree to disagree. For example, you may not see eye to eye on your daughter's choice of clothes or hairstyle, but you should try to accept that it is her choice to make. By approaching conflict calmly and respectfully, parents can help their daughters learn how to resolve conflict in a healthy way, which will serve them well in all of their future relationships.

A key part of parenting a daughter is helping her to develop a positive self-image and a healthy body image. This can be especially challenging during the teenage years, when girls may be faced with unrealistic beauty standards and intense peer pressure. Parents can help by encouraging their daughter's unique strengths and abilities, and by modeling positive self-talk and body image. It is also important to avoid making negative comments about your own body or appearance, as your daughter may internalize these messages. Instead, focus on emphasizing the importance of health and well-being, rather than appearance. If your daughter is struggling with body image issues, it is important to seek professional help and support. With the right support, your daughter can develop a positive self-image that will last a lifetime.

As daughters grow up, they will eventually begin to explore romantic relationships and sexual intimacy. Parents need to have open and honest conversations with their daughters about these topics, even if it feels uncomfortable. The goal is to provide accurate information and to promote safe and healthy choices. It is also important to be supportive and non-judgmental so that your daughter feels comfortable coming to you with any questions or concerns. By having these conversations early and often, you can help your daughter develop a healthy and positive approach to sex and relationships.

As a parent, your ultimate goal is to help your daughter become a confident, successful adult. There are many things you can do to set her up for success, such as providing her with opportunities to explore her interests and passions, encouraging her to set goals and work towards them, and helping her to develop strong time management and organization skills. It is also important to celebrate your daughter's successes, no matter how small, and to offer support and encouragement when she faces challenges. With your support, your daughter will be able to achieve anything she sets her mind to.

Finally, as your daughter grows up, remember to take time to enjoy the journey. There may be difficult times, but also there will be fantastic times of great growth and change. By enjoying the ups and downs, and savouring the special moments, you can create a lasting bond with your daughter that will last a lifetime. And as you watch your daughter blossom into a confident and capable woman, you will know that you have done your job well.

# Chapter 1: How to Communicate with your Daughter

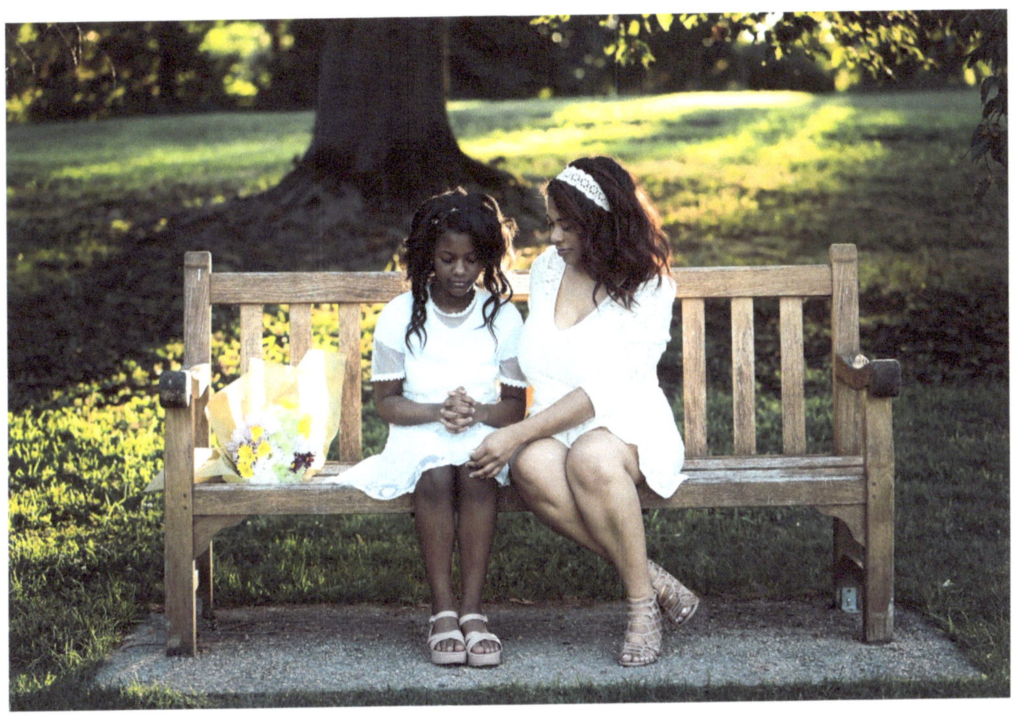

*Figure 2: One of the most important aspects of communication with your daughter is talking about emotions and feelings*

"Communication" is key when it comes to any relationship, but it's especially important when it comes to your relationship with your daughter. As your daughter grows and develops, it's crucial that you can communicate with her in a way that is open, honest, and supportive. In this book, we'll explore some of the best ways to communicate with your daughter, from infancy to adulthood. We'll discuss how to build a strong foundation of trust and respect, and how to adapt your approach as she gets older. With these tools, you can create a lasting and meaningful relationship with your daughter that will benefit both of you for years to come

In this first chapter, we'll start by talking about the importance of communication from a young age. Even when your daughter is a baby, you can start laying the groundwork for open and honest communication. We'll discuss how to use eye contact, body language, and verbal cues to communicate with your daughter in a way that she understands. As she gets older, we'll look at ways to talk to her about more complex topics, like feelings, emotions, and relationships. We'll also discuss the importance of active listening, and how to show your daughter that you're truly hearing what she has to say. By following the tips and advice in this book, you can create a strong, healthy, and loving relationship with your daughter that will last a lifetime.

## The Importance of Listening

As we discussed in the previous chapter, listening is one of the most important parts of communication. When you're listening to your daughter, it's important to give her your full attention and avoid distractions. This means putting down your phone, turning off the TV, and looking her in the eye.

You should also resist the urge to jump in and solve her problems right away. Instead, try to really hear what she's saying, and reflect back what you've heard. This will show her that you're really listening, and it will help her to feel heard and understood. Even if you don't agree with everything she's saying, it's important to validate her feelings and let her know that you care about her. It may not be easy to do, but it will be worth it in the end.

## Talking About Emotions and Feelings

One of the most important aspects of communication with your daughter is talking about emotions and feelings. This can be difficult, but it's important to create a safe space for her to express herself. Start by modelling appropriate ways to talk about emotions. This means using "I" statements, rather than "you" statements, and avoiding criticism and judgment. For example, instead of saying, "You're being so dramatic," you could say, "I'm sensing that you're feeling frustrated." This will help your daughter feel comfortable sharing her feelings with you.

## Setting Boundaries

Another important part of communication is setting boundaries. It's important to be clear and consistent with your boundaries, and to explain the reasons behind them. For example, you could say, "I want to be able to have an open and honest relationship with you, but I'm not comfortable with you sharing graphic details about your relationships. Can we agree on some boundaries around that?" Setting boundaries may be difficult at first, but it's important to stick to them to build trust and respect.

## Dealing with Conflict

No matter how well you communicate, there will be times when you and your daughter disagree. It's important to approach conflict calmly and respectfully. Avoid yelling or name-calling, and try to stay focused on the issue at hand, rather than bringing up past disagreements. You could say something like, "I'd like to talk about this problem without getting upset. Can we start over and try to work through it together?" If your daughter gets angry or starts to escalate the conflict, try to stay calm and remind her that you're on her side. With time and practice, you can learn to resolve conflicts healthily and productively.

## Talking About Difficult Subjects

There may be some topics that are particularly difficult to talk about with your daughter. These could include things like death, sexual assault, drugs, or mental health issues. It's important to approach these subjects with sensitivity and understanding. Start by listening to your daughter and letting her lead the conversation. Try to avoid advising unless she asks for it. Instead, focus on validating her feelings and showing empathy. If you're not sure what to say, you can always ask her how you can be most supportive. Just being there to listen can make a big difference.

## Communicating Through Technology

In today's world, much of our communication happens through technology like texting, social media, and video chat. While these methods of communication can be convenient, they can also present some unique challenges. For example, it can be difficult to convey tone or body language through a text message. To communicate effectively through technology, it's important to be clear and concise. Make sure your messages are easy to understand and avoid using abbreviations or slang that your daughter might not know. It's also important to be respectful of your daughter's boundaries when it comes to technology. If she doesn't want to be contacted after a certain time, respect that boundary.

## Parenting During the Teenage Years

The teenage years can be particularly challenging for both parents and daughters. During this time, your daughter is going through a lot of changes, both physically and emotionally. It's important to be patient and understanding during this time. Try to focus on maintaining a connection with your daughter, even if she is pulling away. It's normal for her to want to spend more time with friends and less time with family during this stage of life. However, it's important to maintain a sense of connection and to continue to communicate with her as much as possible. Even small gestures like a quick text or a short phone call can make a big difference.

## Maintaining a Healthy Relationship

Maintaining a healthy relationship with your daughter is an ongoing process. It takes time, effort, and commitment from both of you. Here are a few things to keep in mind:

- ❖ Be present and involved in your daughter's life.
- ❖ Encourage her interests and passions.
- ❖ Respect her boundaries and give her space.
- ❖ Be a role model for the kind of person you want her to be.
- ❖ Talk to her about the tough stuff, like sex, drugs, and other difficult topics.
- ❖ Don't forget to have fun together!

## Navigating the Changing Landscape of Adolescence

As your daughter grows and changes, it's important to stay informed about the latest research and developments in the field of adolescent development. This will help you to better understand and respond to the changes your daughter is going through. You can find information about adolescent development from a variety of sources, including books, articles, and online resources. By staying informed, you can help your daughter navigate this challenging and exciting time in her life.

## The Importance of Self-Care for Parents

As a parent, it's easy to get so focused on your daughter's needs that you forget to take care of your own. However, it's important to remember that you can't pour from an empty cup. Taking care of your own physical and emotional well-being is crucial to being the best parent you can be. Here are a few ideas for self-care:

- Make time for your hobbies and interests.
- Get enough sleep and exercise.
- Eat a healthy, balanced diet.
- Spend time with friends and family.
- Don't be afraid to ask for help when you need it.

## The Teenage Brain

One of the most important things to understand about your daughter during adolescence is how her brain is developing and changing. The teenage brain goes through a process called pruning, where unneeded neural connections are eliminated. This pruning process is important for the development of the teenage brain, but it can also lead to increased impulsivity and risk-taking behavior. It's important to be aware of these changes so that you can be supportive and understanding of your daughter's behaviour. This knowledge can also help you to set appropriate boundaries and consequences for her behaviour.

## Dealing with Conflict

Conflict is a normal part of any relationship, including the parent-child relationship. When conflict arises, it's important to stay calm and try to see things from your daughter's perspective. Be clear about your boundaries and expectations, but also be willing to listen and compromise. Use "I" statements when you express your needs and feelings, and avoid blaming or criticizing your daughter. Try to find common ground where you can agree, and focus on solutions rather than dwelling on the problem. With patience and practice, you can learn to navigate conflict healthily and productively.

## Building a Positive Parent-Daughter Relationship

Building a positive relationship with your daughter takes time and effort. Start by committing to spend quality time together regularly. This can be anything from having dinner together as a family to taking a walk after school. Whatever you choose, make sure it's something you both enjoy. This will help to strengthen your bond and create a foundation of trust and respect. Also, remember to focus on the positive qualities of your daughter and celebrate her successes, big and small. And most importantly, tell her that you love her.

It's also important to remember that your daughter's behaviour is often a reflection of how she feels about herself. If she is struggling with low self-esteem, it may show up in her behaviour. In these cases, it's especially important to focus on building up her self-confidence and self-worth.

Look for opportunities to help her feel good about herself, and avoid comparing her to others. Instead, focus on her unique strengths and abilities. By doing this, you can help her to develop a healthy self-image and the confidence to face the challenges of adolescence.

## The Impact of Technology on Parent-Daughter Relationships

In today's world, technology plays a major role in our lives, and this is especially true for teenagers. While technology can have many benefits, it can also present challenges for parents and daughters. Social media can be a source of peer pressure and comparison, and it can also lead to cyberbullying. Smartphones and other devices can also interfere with face-to-face communication. Despite these challenges, there are ways to use technology to strengthen your relationship with your daughter. One way is to find activities that you can do together using technology, such as playing online games or watching movies. Another way is to set limits on technology use. This could mean limiting screen time or establishing rules about when and where devices can be used. It's also important to model healthy technology habits, such as putting away your own devices when spending time with your daughter. It's also important to stay informed about the latest apps and trends, so you can have open and honest conversations about technology. By doing this, you can help your daughter develop healthy habits and a healthy relationship with technology.

....

# Chapter 2: Understanding your Daughter's Perspective
## Factors that can Influence your Daughter's Perspective

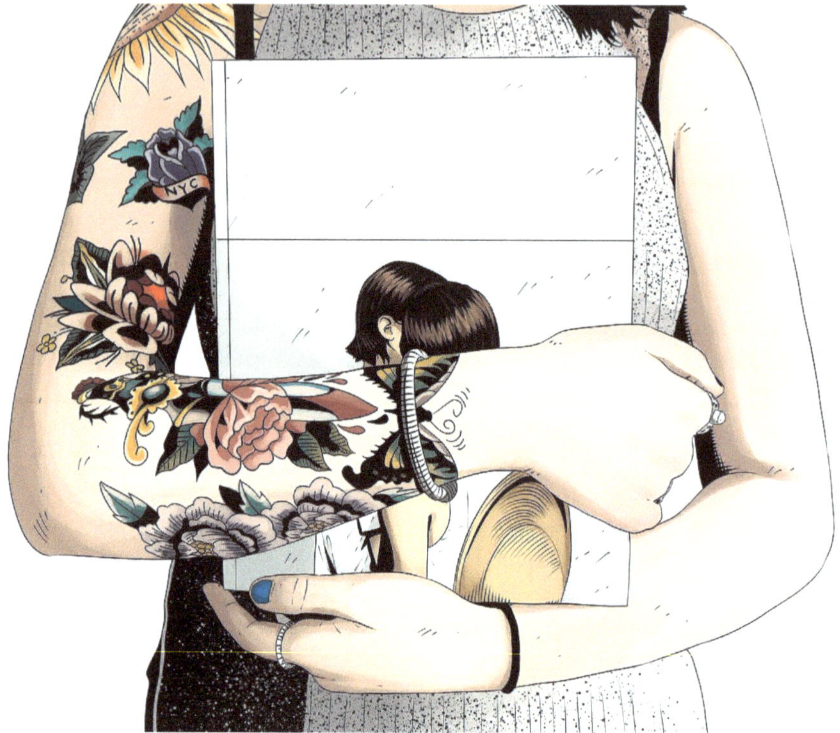

*Figure 3: Another factor that can influence your daughter's perspective is the media and pop culture*

## The Influence of Peers and Groups

One factor that can greatly influence your daughter's perspective is her peer group. During adolescence, peers become increasingly important and can have a major impact on her behaviour, attitudes, and beliefs. While some peer groups can be positive influences, others can be negative, and it's important to understand the difference. Positive peer groups can provide a sense of belonging, acceptance, and support. Negative peer groups, on the other hand, can lead to unhealthy behaviours and risky choices.

## The Role of Media and Pop Culture

Another factor that can influence your daughter's perspective is the media and pop culture. Today's teenagers are constantly bombarded with messages from the media about what they should look like, how they should act, and what is important in life. These messages can be powerful and can lead to unrealistic expectations, low self-esteem, and body image issues. Pop culture can also glamorize unhealthy behaviours, such as substance use, and can perpetuate stereotypes and misinformation. As a parent, it's important to be aware of the messages your daughter is receiving and to provide her with accurate information.

## The Influence of Family Dynamics

Family dynamics also play a significant role in your daughter's perspective. The quality of the parent-child relationship, sibling relationships, and family communication can all have an impact. If your daughter feels loved, accepted, and supported by her family, she is more likely to have a positive self-image and to make healthy choices. On the other hand, if there is conflict, criticism, or negativity in the family, it can have the opposite effect. It's important to foster a loving and supportive home environment and to make time for family bonding.

## The Impact of School and Educational Experiences

Your daughter's school and educational experiences can also have a significant impact on her perspective. The academic environment, the quality of the teachers, and the overall climate of the school can all play a role. Additionally, extracurricular activities and involvement in school can have a positive or negative impact. Research has shown that high-quality extracurricular activities can improve self-esteem and social skills, while involvement in negative or risky activities can have the opposite effect. It's important to encourage your daughter to participate in activities that are positive and healthy.

## The Influence of Religion and Spirituality

Finally, it's important to consider the influence of religion and spirituality on your daughter's perspective. Religious beliefs and practices can have a significant impact on her worldview, values, and self-identity. In some cases, religion can provide a sense of community, support, and meaning. However, in other cases, it can lead to feelings of judgment, exclusion, or even conflict. It's important to respect your daughter's beliefs and to encourage her to explore her spirituality in a healthy and supportive way.

## Conclusion

These are just a few of the many factors that can influence your daughter's perspective. It's important to be aware of these influences and to do your best to provide a supportive and positive environment. Additionally, it's important to recognize that your daughter is an individual and that her perspective may not always align with your own. It's okay to disagree, and it's important to allow her to form her own opinions and beliefs. At the same time, you can provide guidance and support to help her navigate the complex world of adolescence.

...

# Chapter 3: Breaking the Ice: Starting Conversations with your Daughter

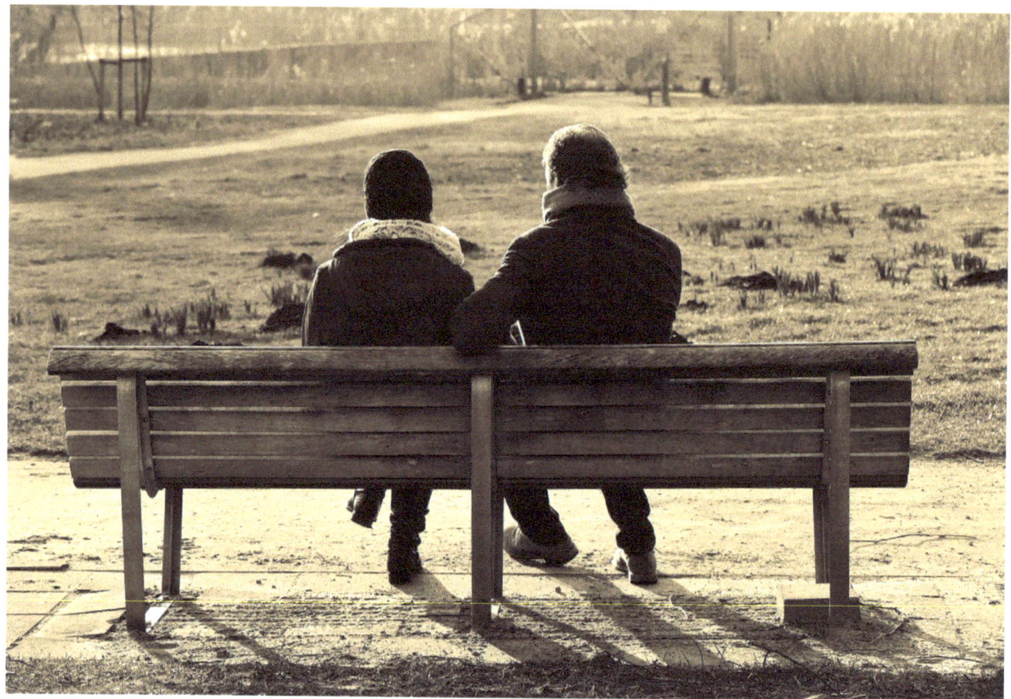

*Figure 4: It's important to find a time when your daughter is relaxed and not distracted by other things to break the ice and start a difficult conversation*

One of the most challenging parts of communicating with your daughter is breaking the ice. Whether you're having a difficult conversation or just trying to make small talk, it can be tough to get the conversation started. In this chapter, we'll explore some strategies for breaking the ice and making the first move. We'll look at things like choosing the right time and place, using open-ended questions, and starting with something light-hearted. By following these tips, you can start your conversations off on the right foot and build a stronger relationship with your daughter.

## Right Time and Place

Let's start by considering the right time and place for starting a conversation. It's important to find a time when your daughter is relaxed and not distracted by other things. For example, if she's just come home from school or practice, she may be feeling tired or stressed. Instead, try to find a time when she's settled in and ready to talk. In terms of place, choose somewhere that is comfortable and free from distractions. This could be the living room, the kitchen, or her bedroom. By choosing the right time and place, you can set the stage for a successful conversation.

## Open-ended Questions

Next, let's talk about using open-ended questions. These are questions that can't be answered with a simple yes or no. For example, instead of asking *"Did you have a good day at school?"* try asking *"What was the best part of your day?".* This type of question allows your daughter to share more about her experience and gives you a chance to dig deeper into the conversation. Open-ended questions can also help to start a conversation about a difficult topic. For example, if you're worried about your daughter's social media use, you could ask "How do you feel about the role of social media in your life?" This type of question allows your daughter to share her thoughts and feelings without feeling judged.

## Using Humour to Break the Ice

Finally, let's talk about using humour to break the ice. Sometimes a little bit of levity can be the perfect way to start a conversation. Try using a light-hearted icebreaker, like telling a joke or sharing a funny story. Humour can help to diffuse tension and put both you and your daughter at ease. Just make sure that your humour is appropriate and in line with your daughter's sense of humour. If you're not sure if a joke will land, try testing it out on someone else first.

## Conclusion

Starting conversations with your daughter doesn't have to be difficult. By choosing the right time and place, using open-ended questions, and employing humour, you can break the ice and start a conversation that is meaningful and productive. Do you have any other tips or strategies for starting conversations with your daughter?

....

# Chapter 4: Talking to your Daughter transitioning to Puberty and Adolescence

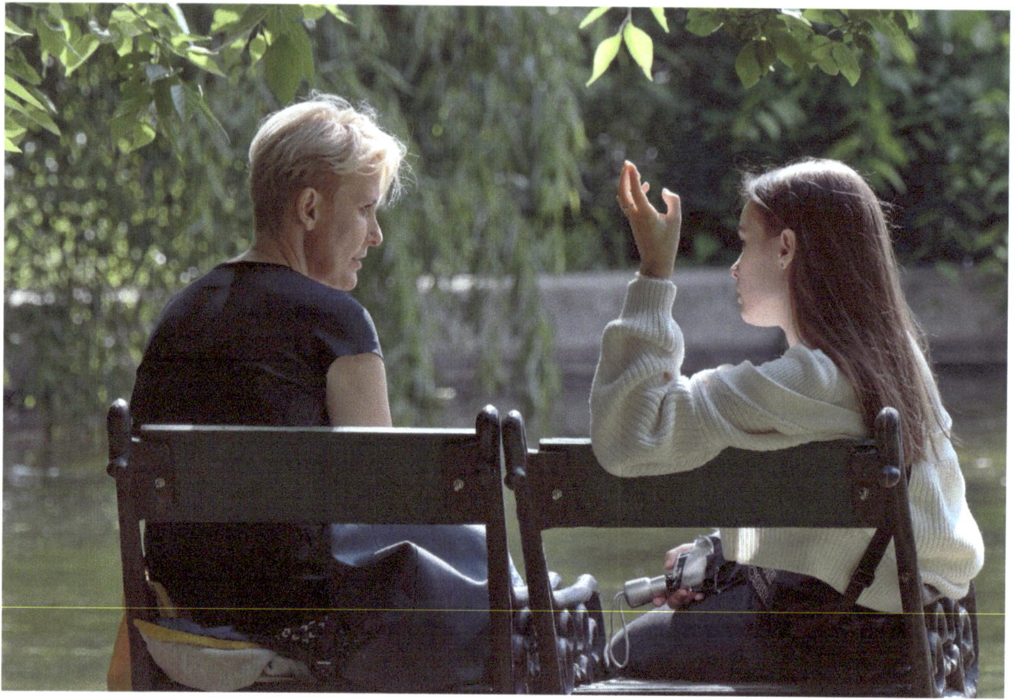

*Figure 5: As a parent, always ensure your Daughter that Puberty is an Awesome experience and as natural as our existence*

There are a lot of myths and misconceptions about puberty and adolescence, and it can be difficult for parents to separate fact from fiction. In this chapter, we'll dispel some of the most common myths, including the idea that puberty is a "rite of passage" that must be endured, that all girls experience the same changes, and that parents don't need to be involved in their daughter's puberty journey. By dispelling these myths, we can help parents and their daughters approach this transition with more confidence and understanding.

## Tell Your Daughter that Puberty is an Awesome Experience

One of the most common myths about puberty is that it's a "rite of passage" that must be endured. In reality, puberty is a natural part of growing up and can be a positive experience. Parents need to provide support and encouragement, rather than treating it as a test of strength or endurance. In addition, each girl's experience of puberty is unique, and not all girls will go through the same physical and emotional changes. Therefore, parents need to avoid comparing their daughter's experience to others. As a parent, always ensure your Daughter that Puberty is an Awesome experience and as natural as our existence.

## Be Involved in Your Daughter's Puberty Journey

Another myth is that parents don't need to be involved in their daughter's puberty journey. Research has shown that when parents are involved, their daughters tend to have a more positive experience of puberty. Parents can help by providing accurate information, setting a good example, and offering emotional support. There are also some practical things parents can do to help their daughters, such as providing a comfortable space to talk about puberty, ensuring that their daughter has easy access to hygiene products, and helping them to develop healthy habits.

In addition to dispelling these myths, parents can also help their daughters understand that there is no "right" or "wrong" way to experience puberty. By focusing on celebrating each girl's unique journey, parents can help their daughters feel more comfortable and confident during this important time.

## Conclusion

Dispelling myths and misconceptions about puberty and adolescence can help parents provide their daughters with the support and information they need to navigate this important time in their lives. By focusing on celebrating each girl's unique journey, parents can help their daughters feel more comfortable and confident.

...

# Chapter 5: Talking to your Daughter about Sex

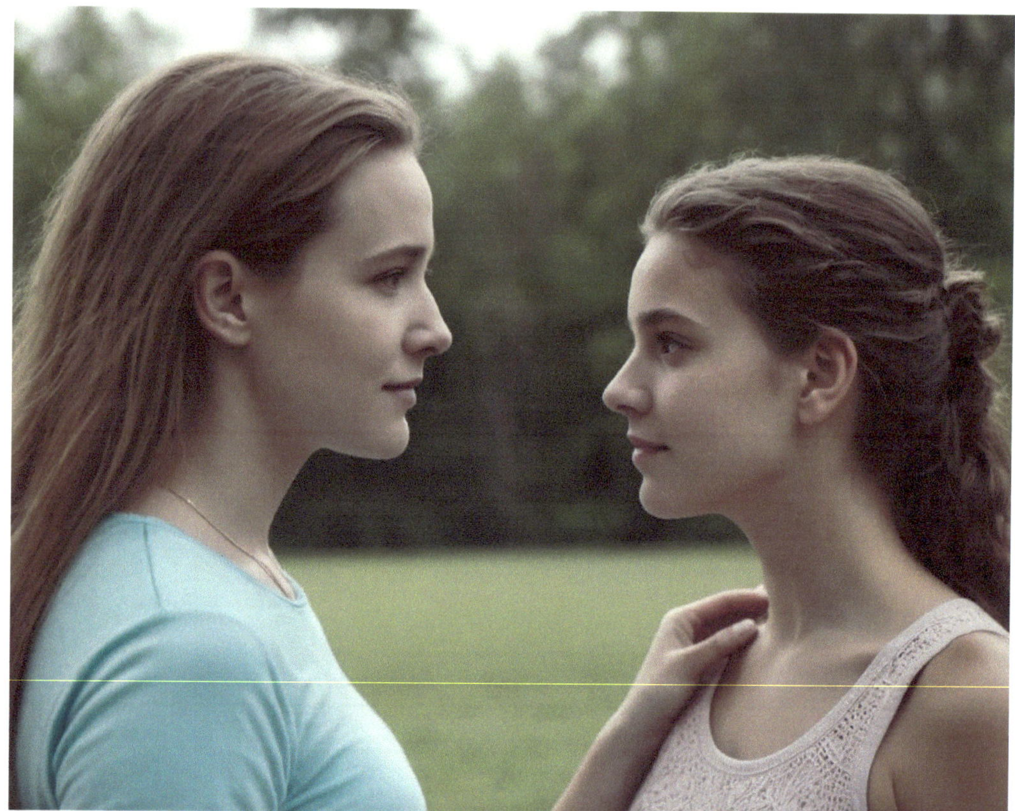

*Figure 6: The first step in talking to your daughter about sex is to make sure you're prepared*

Talking to your daughter about sex can be awkward and uncomfortable, but it's an important part of being a parent. In this chapter, we'll explore how to approach this topic in a way that's both age-appropriate and comfortable for you and your daughter. We'll cover some of the common questions and concerns parents have about talking to their daughters about sex, and provide some tips on how to make the conversation as easy as possible.

## Be Well-Prepared

The first step in talking to your daughter about sex is to make sure you're prepared. This means thinking about what you want to say, how you want to say it, and what you're comfortable with your daughter knowing. It's also important to be aware of your daughter's maturity level and to tailor your conversation accordingly. For example, a younger daughter may only need basic information about the physical changes that occur during puberty, while an older daughter may be ready to learn about more advanced topics like safe sex and consent. Once you've thought about what you want to say, it's time to start the conversation.

## Start the Conversation

It's best to choose a time when you and your daughter are relaxed and have some privacy, like during a car ride or before bedtime. You may also want to frame the conversation in a way that makes it feel more natural, like,

*"I've been thinking about how much you're growing up and how we can talk about some of the changes you're going through."*

Avoid language that is overly clinical or clinical, as this can make the conversation feel awkward or uncomfortable.

You may also want to begin by asking your daughter what she already knows about sex. This will give you a good starting point and help you avoid repeating information she already knows. It's important to answer her questions honestly and directly, without getting embarrassed or sidestepping the issue. If you're not sure how to answer a question, it's okay to say you don't know and offer to find out the answer together. You can also use this opportunity to reinforce the idea that it's okay to talk about sex and that she can always come to you with questions or concerns.

As you answer your daughter's questions, try to use non-judgmental language and avoid making her feel guilty or ashamed.

*For example, instead of saying, "It's not okay for you to have sex," you could say, "We believe that sex is something that should happen in a committed relationship." This type of language is less likely to make your daughter feel bad or embarrassed, and it also allows her to ask more questions if she has them.*

As the conversation progresses, you may want to focus on specific topics like safe sex, STDs, and consent.

It's important to approach these topics in a way that's both factual and supportive. Be honest about the risks of unsafe sex, but don't scare your daughter or make her feel like she's not in control of her own body. Instead, focus on giving her the information she needs to make safe and informed decisions. You can also talk about the emotional side of sex, like the importance of communication and respecting boundaries.

Finally, be sure to discuss consent, which means that both people need to agree to any sexual activity and can change their minds at any time. It's also important to let your daughter know that she can always say no, even if she has said yes in the past.

You may also want to talk about healthy relationships, including what it means to be a good partner and what red flags to look out for. Ultimately, your goal should be to make your daughter feel comfortable and confident about making her own decisions. You want her to know that she can always come to you for information, support, and advice. This will help her build a strong foundation for her future relationships.

## Be Patient and Understanding

As you're having this conversation, remember to be patient and understanding. Your daughter may be nervous or uncomfortable, and that's okay. It's important to give her time to process the information and ask questions. It may also take multiple conversations to cover all of the topics you want to discuss. By taking things slowly and being supportive, you can help your daughter navigate this difficult and sometimes confusing time.

Remember, you don't have to be an expert on everything. You may not know all the answers, and that's okay. You can always find resources to help you and your daughter, like books, websites, and even your daughter's doctor or school ccounselor with the right support and information, you can help your daughter navigate the complicated world of adolescence and build a strong foundation for her future.

## Talk to her about Positive Body Image

One topic that is important to discuss with your daughter is about body image. This can be a difficult and sensitive topic, but it's an important one to address. Many girls struggle with body image issues, especially during their teenage years. You can help your daughter develop a healthy body image by focusing on her strengths and talents, and by modelling positive self-talk. You can also help her find role models who have a healthy body image, and you can avoid making negative comments about your own body or other people's bodies.

When talking to your daughter about body image, it's important to focus on health and wellness, not just appearance. You should emphasize that there is no "right" way to look and that everyone is different. You should also help your daughter understand that the media often portrays unrealistic body standards and that these images are often edited or altered. It's also a good idea to talk to your daughter about the importance of self-care and self-love. These include eating well, exercising, and taking care of your mental health. These are all important aspects of a healthy body image.

## Talk to her about STDs

STDs, or sexually transmitted diseases, are a serious topic that many parents and teens find difficult to discuss. However, it's important to have this conversation early and often. The earlier your daughter understands the risks of STDs and how to protect herself, the better off she'll be.

Do talk about how to prevent the spread of STDs, including using protection and getting tested regularly. By having this conversation, you can help your daughter stay safe and healthy.

Here is some general but very key information you can share about common STDs to watch out for:

a. **HPV (Human papillomavirus)**
   This is one of the most common STDs in most countries in the world. There are over 100 different types of HPV, and some strains can cause cancer. HPV is spread through skin-to-skin contact, and it can be passed even when there are no symptoms. Your daughter needs to understand that anyone sexually active is at risk for HPV, regardless of gender or sexual orientation. There are vaccines available that can help protect against some strains of HPV. If your daughter hasn't been vaccinated yet, talk to her doctor

about whether it's right for her. If your daughter is sexually active, it's also important for her to get tested regularly. Many STDs don't have symptoms, so regular testing is the only way to know for sure if she has been infected. It's also important to talk to your daughter about the importance of using protection. This includes condoms and other barriers, such as dental dams. Using protection is the best way to reduce the risk of getting an STD. Do you have any questions about HPV or other STDs?

b.  **Chlamydia**

Another common STD is chlamydia. This is a bacterial infection that is spread through sexual contact. Chlamydia can cause serious health problems, including infertility if it's not treated. The good news is that chlamydia is easily treated with antibiotics. However, many people don't know they have it, because the symptoms can be mild or even non-existent. This is another reason why regular STD testing is so important. You should also talk to your daughter about the importance of being honest with her partner about her STD status. Being honest is the best way to protect herself and her partner.

c.  **Gonorrhea**

This is another bacterial infection that is spread through sexual contact. Like chlamydia, gonorrhea can cause serious health problems if it's not treated. It's also easy to treat with antibiotics. However, gonorrhea is becoming resistant to some antibiotics, so it's important to get tested and treated as soon as possible. There are also vaccines available that can help protect against certain strains of gonorrhea. It's important to remember that no vaccine is 100% effective, so regular STD testing is still necessary.

d.  **Syphilis**

This is a bacterial infection that can be spread through sexual contact. Syphilis can cause serious health problems, including blindness, heart disease, and even death. In its early stages, syphilis can be cured with antibiotics. However, if it's not caught and treated early, the damage can be permanent. Syphilis is also becoming resistant to some antibiotics, so it's important to get tested and treated as soon as possible. Your daughter should also know that condoms are not 100% effective at preventing syphilis, so regular STD testing is still necessary.

e.  **Herpes**

This is a viral infection that can be spread through sexual contact. There are two types of herpes: HSV-1 and HSV-2. HSV-1 is most commonly associated with cold sores, while HSV-2 is most commonly associated with genital herpes. Both types can cause genital herpes, but most people with herpes don't have any symptoms. There is no cure for herpes, but there are medications that can help manage the symptoms. It's important to get tested for herpes if you have any symptoms, even if they are mild. This is because you can still spread the virus even if you don't have symptoms.

f.  **HIV**

One final STD that we should discuss is HIV. This is a virus that attacks the immune system. If left untreated, HIV can lead to AIDS. However, there are effective treatments for HIV that can help people live long and healthy lives. Your daughter needs to know that there is no cure for HIV, but there are ways to prevent it. The best way to prevent HIV is to use protection, get tested regularly, and know the status of your partner.

....

# Chapter 6: Talking to your Daughter about Sexual Consent

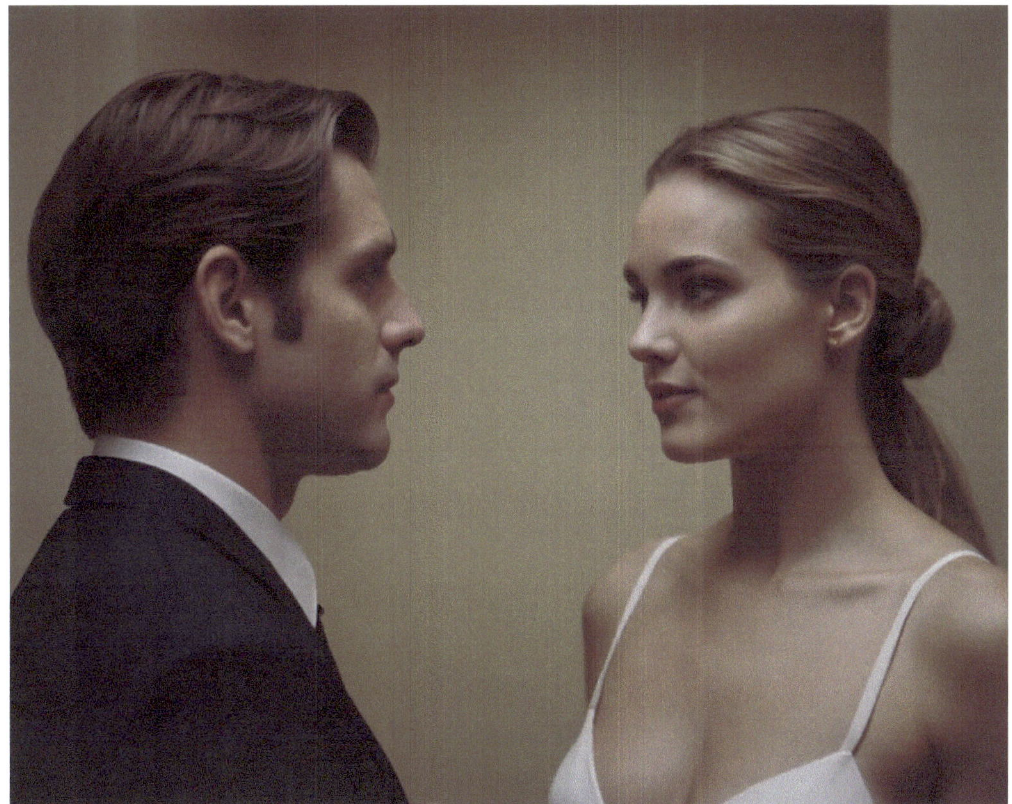

*Figure 7: Consent must be given freely and without coercion. Teach your daughter about this*

Sexual consent is about making sure everyone involved in a sexual situation is giving their full, informed, and enthusiastic agreement. This means that everyone involved should be able to understand what they're agreeing to, and they should feel free to say no at any time. This applies to people of all genders, and it's important to teach your daughter about consent from an early age. This way, she'll know how to recognize and respect other people's boundaries, and she'll be able to set her boundaries as well.

## Consent is also an ongoing process, not a one-time event

Just because someone said yes once, it doesn't mean they're automatically agreeing to any future sexual activity. People are also allowed to change their minds at any time, and it's important to respect that.

## Silence is Not Consent

It's also worth noting that silence is not consent. Just because someone doesn't say no, it doesn't mean they're giving their consent.

## When Under Influence of Alcohol or Drugs, No Consent

Lastly, someone can't give consent if they're under the influence of drugs or alcohol. Consent must be given freely and without coercion. Teach your daughter about this.

## Why Sexual Consent is Important?

As a parent, it's your job to talk to your daughter about what constitutes sexual consent and why it's so important. This is a difficult conversation to have, but it's a necessary one. You should also talk to your daughter about the consequences of not getting or giving consent. These can include legal consequences, as well as emotional and physical consequences. It's also important to talk to your daughter about what to do if she or someone she knows is the victim of sexual assault. This includes where to go for help and how to get support. By having these difficult conversations, you can help your daughter understand consent and make informed choices about her sexual health.

In addition to sexual consent, it's important to talk to your daughter about other aspects of sexual health, healthy relationships, and boundaries. These are all complex and sensitive topics, but it's better to have these conversations early and often. By doing so, you can help your daughter develop a healthy and positive view of herself and her sexuality.

## Talking to your Daughter about Healthy Relationships

When talking to your daughter about healthy relationships, it's important to start by establishing what makes a relationship healthy. This includes things like mutual respect, trust, and open communication. You should also teach your daughter to recognize the signs of an unhealthy or abusive relationship. These can include jealousy, control, or verbal abuse. It's also important to teach your daughter that she doesn't have to stay in a relationship that's not healthy or safe. She has the right to end a relationship at any time, no matter what. Finally, you should teach your daughter that it's okay to ask for help if she needs it.

## Talking to your Daughter about the Importance of Boundaries

 Boundaries are the limits that a person sets for themselves and others. They can be physical, emotional, or sexual. It's important to teach your daughter that she has the right to set boundaries and that she doesn't have to compromise her comfort or safety for someone else. You should also teach your daughter how to recognize when someone else is violating her boundaries. It's also important to teach your daughter how to respond when someone is violating her boundaries.

One way to approach this topic is to use the concept of "the three Ps": polite, persistent, and physical. When someone is violating your daughter's boundaries, she should first try to be polite and explain why the behaviour is not okay. If the person doesn't listen, she should be persistent and continue to assert her boundaries. Finally, if the person still doesn't listen, she should remove herself from the situation physically. This could mean walking away, leaving the room, or even leaving the house. By teaching your daughter about the three Ps, you can help her stay safe and protect her boundaries.

....

# Chapter 7: Empowering your Daughter

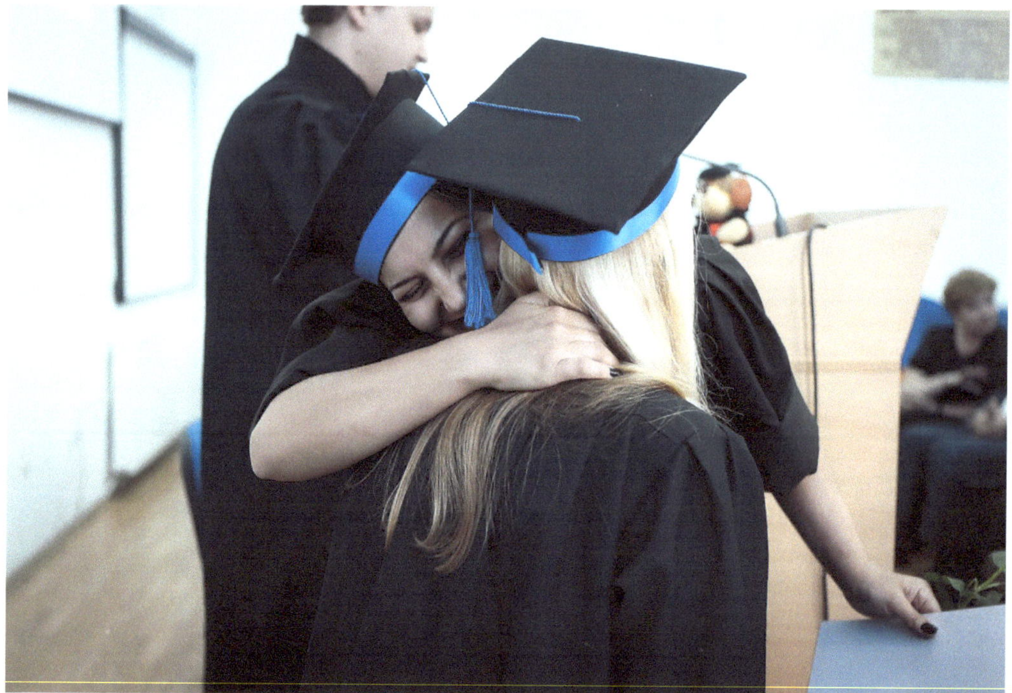

*Figure 8: Empowering your daughter is about more than just teaching her how to be confident and successful.*

Empowering your daughter is about more than just teaching her how to be confident and successful. It's also about teaching her to stand up for herself and others. One thing that's important to remember is that empowerment is not a one-time event. It's a process that takes time and effort. You may not see results right away, but you're planting the seeds for a strong and confident young woman. The best thing you can do is to be there for your daughter, and to encourage her to be her best self.

## Model Respectful Behaviour Yourself

One way to empower your daughter is to model respectful behavior yourself. This means treating your daughter and others with respect and setting a good example of how to treat others fairly. As old wisdom teaches us you gain respect from others by respecting them; when your daughter learns to respect others, she will become a respected member of the community herself.

## Encourage her to Express Herself Freely

You should encourage your daughter to speak up for herself, and to stand up for what she believes in. This could be anything from advocating for herself in school to standing up for a friend who is being bullied. The biggest indicator of an empowered lady, is the ability for one to express herself freely and stand for what she believes in.

## Help her find her Passion

This could be anything from art to science to sports. Encouraging your daughter to pursue her interests can help her develop a strong sense of self and confidence. It can also give her the skills and knowledge she needs to succeed in life. It's important to remember that your daughter's passions may change over time, and that's okay. You should encourage her to explore different interests and find what makes her feel happy and fulfilled.

## Respect her Voice and Opinions

In addition to finding her passion, your daughter needs to feel like she has a voice and is heard. This means listening to her when she talks and taking her concerns seriously. It's also important to show her that her opinion matters by asking for her input and including her in decisions. For example, if you're planning a family trip, you could ask your daughter to help choose the destination. Or, if you're making a major purchase, you could ask her opinion on what you should buy. Giving your daughter a voice will help her feel like she has power and control over her own life.

## Assure her that she is Strong and Capable

Finally, it's important to teach your daughter that she is strong and capable. This means encouraging her to try new things, even if she's afraid. You can also help her learn to problem-solve and overcome challenges. You can do this by modeling a growth mindset and helping her see failure as an opportunity to learn and grow. For example, if your daughter is struggling with a particular school subject, you could help her develop strategies for overcoming this challenge. You could also praise her effort, rather than just her results. By teaching your daughter that she is strong and capable, you can help her develop resilience and confidence.

## Model a Positive Body Image

Another important aspect of empowering your daughter is to model a positive body image yourself. This means being comfortable in your skin, and not putting too much emphasis on physical appearance. It also means avoiding negative body talk, both about yourself and others. Your daughter will learn.

## Empower your Daughter Financially

Empowering your daughter financially is about much more than simply teaching her to save money or invest wisely. It's also about teaching her to feel confident and capable when it comes to money matters. Here are some ideas for empowering your daughter financially:

- Help her develop a strong work ethic. This can include encouraging her to pursue her passions and teaching her the importance of earning an income.
- Talk openly and honestly about money matters. This includes discussing things like budgets, savings goals, and the difference between wants and needs.
- Encourage her to take charge of her finances. This could include giving her an allowance or helping her open her bank account. You could also teach her about things like interest rates, compound interest, and other financial concepts.
- Talk to her about credit and debt. This includes helping her understand the benefits and risks of credit cards and loans. You should also talk about the importance of maintaining a good credit score.
- Encourage her to donate some of her money to a cause she believes in. This can help her learn about the power of money to do well in the world.
- Be a role model when it comes to financial responsibility. This includes practicing good financial habits, like paying bills on time and living within your means. You should also avoid overspending or other financial behaviours that could be harmful.

By empowering your daughter financially, you're giving her the tools she needs to be successful in life. You're also teaching her to be responsible and confident when it comes to money matters. She'll be able to make informed decisions about her finances and will be less likely to fall into debt or make poor financial choices. You're also allowing her to develop important life skills, like budgeting and saving.

...

# Chapter 8: Talking to your Daughter about Sexual Abuse, Pornography, and Sexual Assault

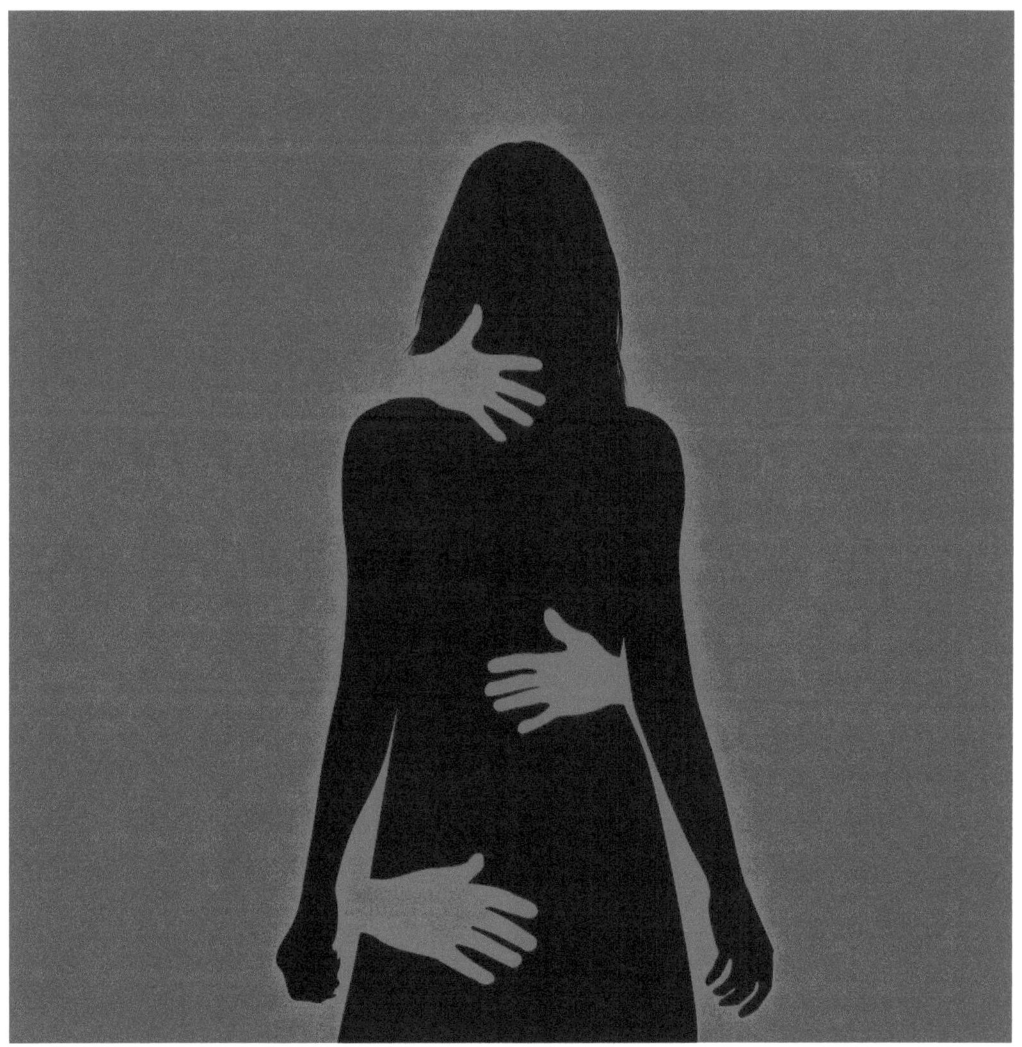

*Figure 9: It's important to teach your daughter how to get help if she's ever in a situation where she feels threatened or unsafe*

Talking to your daughter about sexual abuse, pornography, and sexual assault is difficult, but it's a necessary conversation. These are all serious issues that can have a lasting impact on your daughter's life. It's important to approach these topics in an age-appropriate way and to make sure your daughter knows she can always come to you for help. Here are some tips for having these difficult conversations:

- ❖ Start by asking your daughter if she has any questions about these topics. If she does, answer her questions honestly and without judgment.

- ❖ Be clear about what constitutes sexual abuse, pornography, and sexual assault. This includes defining these terms and providing examples. You should also make it clear that your daughter has the right to say no to any sexual activity, and that no one has the right to pressure her into anything she doesn't want to do.
- ❖ Talk about ways to stay safe. This includes discussing topics like consent, boundaries, and what to do if she feels unsafe. It's also important to teach your daughter how to get help if she's ever in a situation where she feels threatened or unsafe.
- ❖ Help your daughter understand that if she's ever a victim of sexual abuse, it's not her fault. Let her know that you'll always be there to support her and that she can always come to you for help. Reassure her that she won't be in trouble if she tells you about something that's happened to her. It's also important to tell your daughter that she can get help from other trusted adults, like a teacher, doctor, or counselor.
- ❖ Finally, make sure your daughter knows that she can talk to you about anything, no matter how difficult it may be. Show her that you're a safe person to talk to and that you'll listen without judgment.

These conversations may be difficult, but they're an important part of your daughter's development. By having these conversations, you can help your daughter stay safe and make good decisions. You can also give her the tools she needs to feel confident and empowered. It's important to remember that your daughter is growing up in a world where she'll be exposed to a lot of information about sex and sexuality. By talking to her about these topics, you can help her develop a healthy understanding of herself and her body.

## Talking to your Daughter about Online Safety

Another concern that many parents have is how to talk to their daughters about online safety, including issues like cyberbullying and online predators. These are important topics to discuss, and there are a few things you can do to help your daughter stay safe online:

- ❖ Talk to your daughter about what she's doing online, and what sites and apps she's using.
- ❖ Explain the importance of online safety, including not sharing personal information with strangers and being careful about who she talks to online.
- ❖ Set boundaries around screen time, and make sure your daughter understands that she needs to take breaks from screens.
- ❖ Encourage your daughter to come to you if she ever experiences any type of online harassment or bullying. Make sure she knows that she can talk to you about anything, no matter what. It's also a good idea to educate yourself about the latest online safety tools and resources, so you can help your daughter stay safe.

*"Remember, it's not enough to just talk to your daughter about online safety. You also need to model healthy online habits and make sure your online presence is positive and respectful. This will help your daughter learn by example.*

## Talking to your Daughter about the Dangers of Pornography

Having a conversation with your daughter about pornography can be difficult, but it's a necessary part of helping her develop a healthy view of sexuality. It's important to talk to your daughter about pornography in an age-appropriate way and to make sure you're using accurate and honest information.

Here are a few things to keep in mind:

- ❖ First, it's important to have an open and honest conversation with your daughter about sexuality in general. This will help lay the groundwork for a conversation about pornography.
- ❖ Next, make sure you're using accurate and appropriate language when talking about pornography. Don't use words that may be embarrassing or confusing for your daughter.
- ❖ Be sure to answer any questions your daughter has honestly and directly. Avoid getting defensive or upset, even if the topic is difficult. Your daughter needs to know that she can come to you with any question, no matter what.
- ❖ Finally, it's important to talk to your daughter about the potential negative effects of pornography. This includes issues like objectification, unrealistic expectations, and addiction. However, it's also important to acknowledge that not all pornography is harmful and that some people find it enjoyable and empowering.

The goal of this conversation is to help your daughter understand the difference between healthy and unhealthy depictions of sexuality and to make sure she knows that she can come to you with any questions or concerns.

Now, let's talk about some of the most common questions parents have about talking to their daughters about pornography.

*First, at what age should I start talking to my daughter about pornography?*

This is a difficult question, and the answer will vary depending on your daughter's maturity level. However, the American Academy of Paediatrics recommends starting this conversation when your daughter is around 11 or 12 years old. This is the age when many children begin to be exposed to pornography, either accidentally or on purpose.

Next, what should I say to my daughter if she asks me about pornography?

If your daughter asks you about pornography, it's important to be honest and direct. Start by asking your daughter what she already knows about pornography. This will help you tailor your response to her level of understanding. It's also important to let your daughter know that there is no such thing as a "stupid" question and that you're always available to talk to her about anything.

Finally, don't be afraid to use this as an opportunity to discuss your family's values and beliefs about sexuality. This includes topics like consent, respect, and body image. By addressing these issues, you can help your daughter develop a healthy and positive view of sexuality.

## What if my daughter says she's already seen pornography?

If your daughter tells you that she's already seen pornography, don't panic. It's a common experience for children and teenagers, and it doesn't necessarily mean that your daughter has been exposed to anything inappropriate. Instead, use this as an opportunity to have an open and honest conversation with your daughter about what she saw, and how it made her feel.

You can also use this as an opportunity to talk to your daughter about the potential risks of pornography.

# Chapter 9: Sex Education in Schools

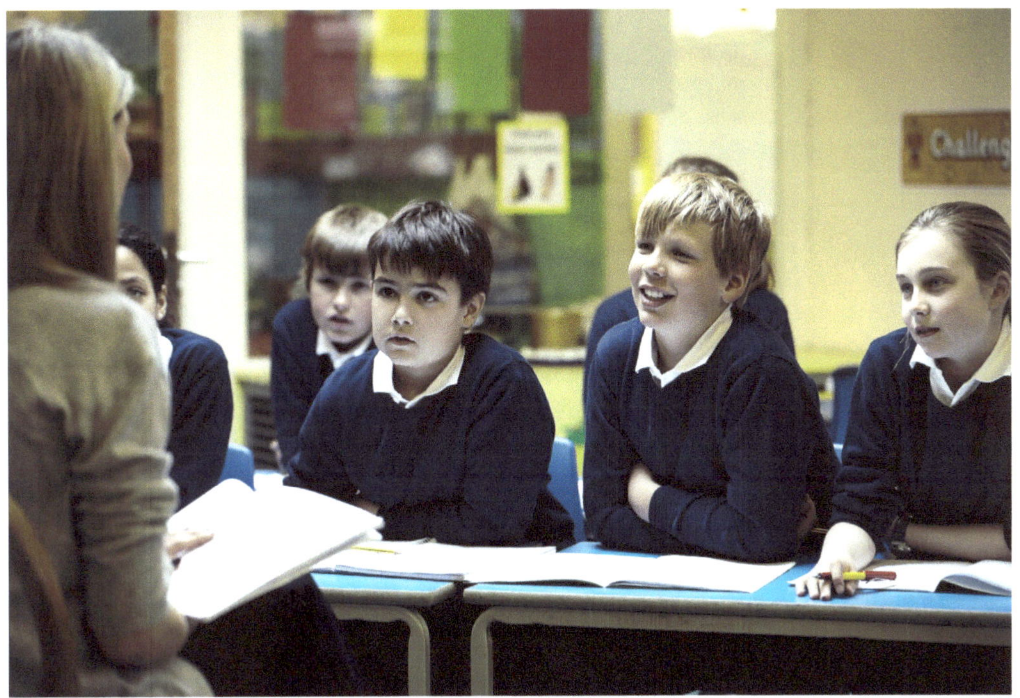

*Figure 10: The goal of sex education is to provide students with accurate and age-appropriate information about sexuality, reproduction, and relationships*

Sex education in schools has been a controversial topic for decades. There is a wide range of views on the subject and a variety of approaches to sex education. Some schools focus on abstinence-only education, while others take a more comprehensive approach. Regardless of the approach, there is a growing consensus that sex education is an important part of a child's overall education.

The goal of sex education is to provide students with accurate and age-appropriate information about sexuality, reproduction, and relationships. This information should be presented in a non-judgmental and supportive environment. It's also important to encourage students to ask questions and to seek out additional information if they need it.

There are a variety of approaches to sex education, and the curriculum varies from state to state. Some states have strict guidelines on what is taught, while others give schools more flexibility. In general, however, the curriculum focuses on topics such as the reproductive system, sexual health, and sexually transmitted infections. Some states also include information on relationships, consent, and sexual orientation. In addition, many schools offer instruction on how to prevent pregnancy and sexually transmitted infections.

However, not all schools offer comprehensive sex education. Many schools do not offer any formal instruction on the subject. This can leave students without the information they need to make informed decisions about their health and sexuality.

There are several challenges associated with sex education in schools. First, it can be difficult to find the right balance between providing accurate information and avoiding controversy. In addition, many parents have strong opinions about what should and should not be taught in the classroom. This can make it difficult for schools to develop a curriculum that is both effective and respectful of different viewpoints.

Finally, there is often a lack of resources and training for teachers who are tasked with delivering sex education. Despite these challenges, there is a growing movement to improve sex education in schools. One way that schools are working to improve sex education is by including more diverse perspectives. For example, some schools are incorporating the perspectives of people with disabilities. This can help students to understand the experiences of others and to develop a more well-rounded understanding of sexuality.

Another way that schools are improving sex education is by using new technologies. For example, some schools are using interactive computer programs to help students learn about sexual health. These programs can be customized to meet the needs of different students, and they can be accessed at any time. This allows students to learn at their own pace and to explore topics that they might not feel comfortable discussing in a classroom setting.

Despite the challenges, sex education is an important part of a child's overall education. By providing students with accurate and comprehensive information, schools can help them to make informed decisions about their health and sexuality. In addition, sex education can help to promote healthy relationships and reduce the risk of sexual violence. Ultimately, a well-rounded and effective sex education curriculum can have a positive impact on the lives of students.

# Chapter 10: Maintaining a Strong and Positive Relationship with your Daughter

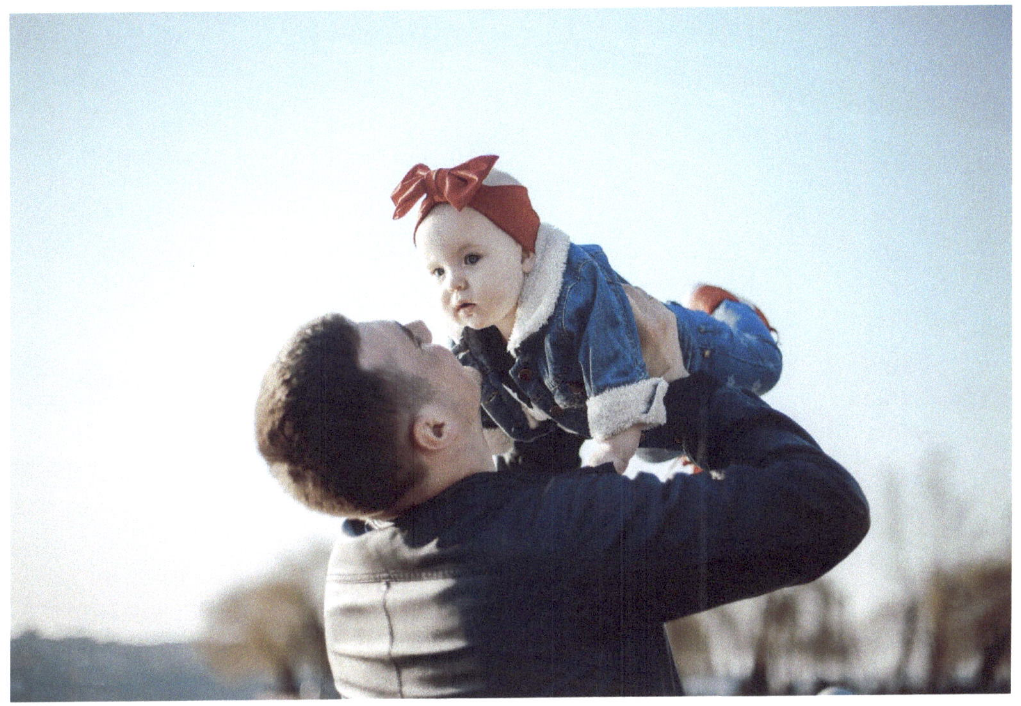

*Figure 11: One of the most important things you can do for your daughter is to be available and present in her life from baby stage to adulthood*

Building a strong and positive relationship with your daughter is an important part of parenting. It takes time, effort, and a lot of love, but it is worth it. Here are some ways to build and maintain a strong relationship with your daughter:

- ❖ Be available and present: One of the most important things you can do for your daughter is to be available and present in her life. This means making time to spend with her, and listening to her when she talks. It also means being there for her when she needs you, whether she's happy or sad.
- ❖ Respect her: It is important to show your daughter respect by listening to her, and by not trying to control her. She is her person, and she deserves to be treated as such. You should also make sure that you're not being overbearing or smothering her. Instead, give her the space she needs to be herself.
- ❖ Set boundaries: Setting boundaries is another important part of building a strong relationship with your daughter. Boundaries are important because they help to create a sense of security and stability. They also help to prevent conflict and misunderstandings. For example, you might set a boundary around bedtime, or around screen time.
- ❖ Show affection: Showing affection is a great way to strengthen your relationship with your daughter. This can be done in many ways, such as hugging her, telling her that you

love her, or doing something special for her. When you show affection, it will help your daughter feel loved and appreciated.

❖ Encourage her interests: Encouraging your daughter's interests is another great way to build a strong relationship with her. This means supporting her passions, even if they're different from your own. For example, if your daughter loves to play sports, you should try to go to her games. Or, if she loves to read, you could take her to the library. Showing interest in your daughter's passions will make her feel valued and supported.

❖ Give her space: It's important to give your daughter space to be herself. This means allowing her to make her own decisions, and not trying to control her life. It is okay to offer guidance and advice, but it's important to let her make her own choices. This will help her to feel independent and capable.

❖ Have fun together: Having fun together is one of the best ways to build a strong relationship with your daughter. This can be anything from going on a trip to playing a game, to simply spending time together. When you have fun together, you'll create memories that will last a lifetime. It's also a great way to build a strong bond.

In addition to these tips, it's also important to lead by example. Be the kind of person you want your daughter to be. Show her what it means to be a good person and a good parent. Be someone that she can look up to and admire. This will help her to become a well-rounded, confident, and successful person.

# Chapter 11: Relating to your Daughter who has now reached Adulthood

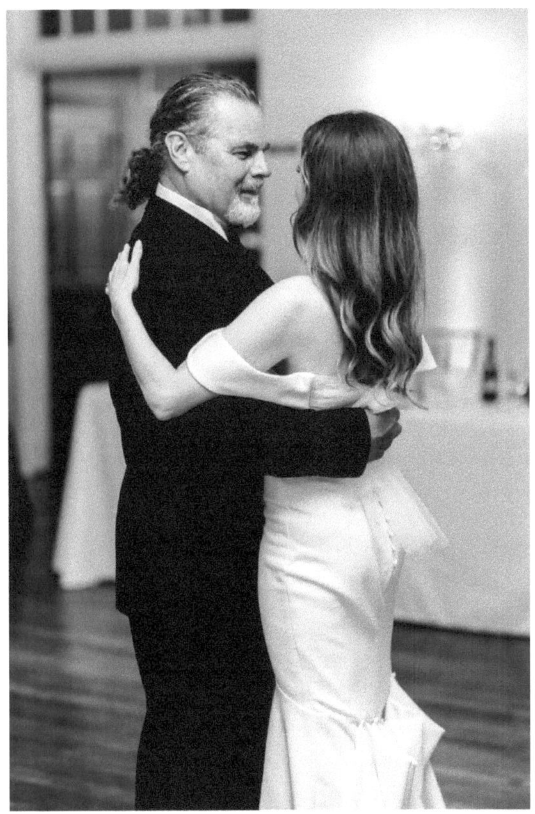

*Figure 12: Your relationship doesn't have to end just because your daughter is becoming an adult. It just means that your role will change.*

As your daughter grows into adulthood, the nature of your relationship will change. She'll be growing more independent and making her own choices, which can be difficult for both of you. But it's important to remember that your relationship doesn't have to end just because she's becoming an adult. It just means that your role will change. Here are some tips for relating to your adult daughter:

- ❖ Give her space: As your daughter becomes an adult, she'll want to have more independence and autonomy. It's important to give her the space she needs to make her own choices and live her own life. Don't try to control her or tell her what to do. Instead, offer support and guidance when she needs it. This will show her that you respect her as an adult.

- ❖ Show interest in her life: Just because your daughter is an adult, that doesn't mean you should stop being interested in her life. Ask her about her job, her friends, her hobbies, and her interests. Let her know that you're still there for her and that you care about what's going on in her life.

- ❖ Respect her boundaries: Just as you need to give your daughter space, you also need to respect her boundaries. If she doesn't want to talk about something, or if she doesn't want you to get involved in a certain situation, you need to respect that. This will show her that you trust her to make her own decisions.
- ❖ Offer advice, but don't push it: As your daughter becomes an adult, she'll likely come to you for advice. But it's important to remember that you're not there to tell her what to do. Offer your perspective and share your experiences, but don't try to force her to do anything. She'll appreciate your honesty and advice more if she knows that you're not trying to control her.
- ❖ Show her unconditional love: No matter what happens, it's important to show your daughter that you love her unconditionally. This means loving her for who she is, not just for what she does. Even if you disagree with her choices, or if she makes mistakes, remind her that you'll always love her. This will help her to feel secure and confident in your relationship.

By following these tips, you can help to create a strong and loving relationship with your adult daughter. This will be a relationship that will last a lifetime. And it will be a source of support and comfort for both of you.

Throughout the different stages of a daughter's life, her relationship with her parents will change. In the early adult years, she may be focused on her independence and establishing her own identity. During this time, she may not want to spend as much time with her parents, or she may feel like she doesn't need them as much. However, it's important to remember that she's still developing and growing and that she'll always need the support of her parents.

As she enters her 30s and 40s, she may start to feel more settled and secure in her life. She may also begin to value her relationship with her parents more and want to spend more time with them. She may also seek out her parents' advice and guidance on a variety of topics, such as career, relationships, and parenting. Parents need to be available and supportive during this stage, but also give their daughter the space she needs to live her own life.

In the later years of adulthood, a daughter may face new challenges, such as caring for aging parents or dealing with mid-life transitions. During this time, a daughter may rely on her parents for more emotional support and guidance. She may also want to spend more time with them, to create memories and strengthen the bond between them. Parents need to be patient and understanding during this stage and listen to their daughter's concerns and needs. It's also important to be realistic about what you can and cannot do for her. You should encourage her to seek professional help when needed.

.....

# Chapter 12: When Daughters become Parents to their Parents

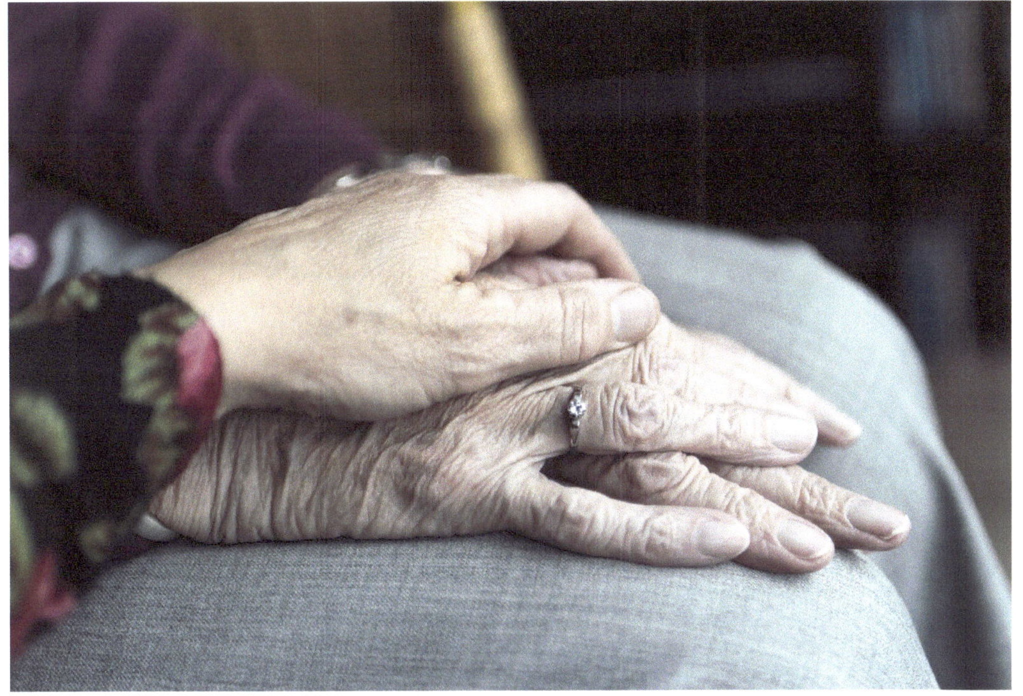

*Figure 13: One of the biggest challenges of taking care of aging parents is dealing with the emotional aspect*

As parents get older, their needs may change. They may need more help with everyday tasks, or they may need more emotional support. No matter what the circumstances, it's important to be prepared to take care of your aging parents. This can be a difficult and emotional process, but there are some things you can do to make it easier. Here are some tips for taking care of your aging parents:

- ❖ Plan ahead: Talk to your parents about their plans, and make sure they have all the necessary legal documents in place. This includes a will, a power of attorney, and a health care proxy.
- ❖ Stay involved: Even if you don't live close to your parents, it's important to stay in touch and check in on them regularly. This can be done through phone calls, video chats, or visits.
- ❖ Be patient: Taking care of an aging parent can be stressful, and it's important to take care of yourself as well. Make sure to schedule time for yourself, and don't be afraid to ask for help.
- ❖ Get support: There are many resources available for people who are taking care of aging parents. This includes support groups, respite care, and in-home care.

Some common concerns include finances, health care decisions, and long-term care planning. It's important to address these concerns as early as possible, so you can make the best decisions for your parents. Do you feel comfortable discussing these issues with your parents?

One of the biggest challenges of taking care of aging parents is dealing with the emotional aspect. It can be difficult to see your parents getting older, and it can be hard to watch them struggle with physical or mental health issues. It's important to remember that it's okay to feel sad or overwhelmed. You can't be expected to be a perfect caregiver, and it's okay to make mistakes. The most important thing is to stay connected to your parents and provide the best care you can. Do you have any concerns about the emotional side of taking care of your aging parents?

Another common concern is balancing your own needs with the needs of your aging parents. It's important to take care of yourself, so you can be the best caregiver possible. This means making time for yourself, and not feeling guilty about it. You may feel like you need to do everything for your parents, but it's important to set boundaries and prioritize your own needs. Have you had any difficulty balancing your needs with the needs of your parents?

As your parents get older, you may need to make decisions about their living situation. This can be a difficult and emotional process, but it's important to consider all the options. Some parents may be able to stay in their own homes with some assistance, while others may need to move into a different living situation. When making these decisions, it's important to take into account your parents' wishes, as well as their physical and mental health. Are you comfortable discussing living arrangements with your parents?

One of the most challenging aspects of taking care of aging parents is navigating the financial side. There are many financial decisions to be made, such as paying for health care, making sure bills are paid, and dealing with legal issues. It's important to get as much information as possible and to seek out professional help when necessary. Do you have any concerns about the financial aspect of taking care of your parents?

One of the best things you can do for your aging parents is to help them stay active and engaged. This can include helping them find activities they enjoy and making sure they stay connected to friends and family. It's also important to help them maintain a sense of independence and control over their lives. Are you doing anything to help your parents stay active and engaged?

...

# BOOK CONCLUSION

Throughout all of these stages, the most important thing is to show your daughter that you love her unconditionally and that you'll always be there for her. It's important to remember that every relationship is unique and that the stages may not always follow this pattern. It's also important to take your daughter's personality and experiences into account. The most important thing is to focus on building a strong and loving relationship, no matter what stage you're in.